How to Look 20 Years Younger Than Your Age

By

Okongor Ayuk Ndifon

Usage:

You may use this ebook without giving it out and without selling it.

DISCLAIMER AND/OR LEGAL NOTICES:

The information presented herein represents author's view as of the date of publication. Due to the fact that the rate with which conditions change, with the use of the internet, the author reserves the right to alter and update his opinion based on the new conditions. It is hoped that the knowledge gained from this ebook would go along way to helping you adapt to the changing condition of the internet.

The ebook is for information purposes only. While every attempt has been made to verify the information provided in this ebook, the author assume any responsibility for errors, wrong interpretation, or omissions. Any slights of people or organizations are unintentional.

The purchaser or reader of this information is responsible for the use of this material, and there is no guarantee of success.

If advice concerning legal or matters related to this material is needed, the services of a fully qualified professional should be sought.

Contents

Introduction

This ebook provides information on how to look 20 years younger than your age, and even look more beautiful.

Most people desire to have a younger looking and beautiful skin, but they think that it is impossible to get such results through some effort.

Youthfulness is achievable when you do some little things expected of you to do as a human. You can not change who you are to become someone else, but with your potential abilities and information, you can become beautiful and younger looking than your age.

It is easy to look up to 20 years younger and more beautiful in six months and friends are sure to sit up and take note, if you take conscious effort and follow the outlined guide below.

1. Secret Steps to Look Younger

The following simple steps to look 20 years younger, would aid you achieve this goal.

1.   Boost your Energy

You energy level may be low, and this makes it impossible to face simple daily challenges that may confront you. When your energy level is low, your energy drops. In order to boost your energy level, you have to ensure that you do everything possible to keep afloat.

2.   Daily Observe Proper Natural Deep Breathing

Make sure that you take adequate amounts of fresh air daily and perform natural deep breathing exercise. Natural deep breathing exercise can be done by breathing from your lower abdomen, inhaling slowly until your lungs are fully expanded, and then exhaling slowly after the count of ten, with your mouth open.

This will enable you to take in enough of fresh air, which is in turn supplied to all your body cells to help you look 20 years younger.

3.   Have Siesta and Catnaps for Five Minutes Daily

You must have a daily siesta of about one hour, to enable you refresh your brain and energy. In addition to a one hour daily siesta, add a five minutes catnap, to enable you get refreshed at all times.

4.   Shed Excess weight

Over-weight is the cause of many health problems; therefore make sure that you cut down your weight if you have excess weight or if you are obese. Obesity can cause you diabetes and other problems.

7

5.   Restore muscle Tone through Physical Exercise

Physical exercise is very important. So, you must engage in daily and regular exercise. You can exercise for 30 to 60 minutes daily, indoors and outdoors.

You can do walking, jogging, swimming, dancing, bicycle riding, stretching of your body, facial exercise, etc. daily. This will tone your muscles and help you look 20 years younger.

6. Eat Balanced Diets

Eating balanced diets on a daily basis would ensure that you have a complete supply of all nutrients, vitamins and minerals. Make sure you get adequate vitamins and minerals by eating whole grains, fish instead of meat, peanut, almonds, cashew nuts, fruits and vegetables, daily.

Do not skip breakfast, because breakfast would help boost your energy from start, by providing all the strength and power to carry you through the day. In your diets, avoid white sugar, but go for honey.

7.   Take Multivitamins Supplements

When your diets are lacking or because of destruction of vitamins and minerals during cooking, add multivitamins capsule or tablets to your meal, to supplement for missing vitamins and minerals.

Make sure that you consume magnesium daily, to enable you do physical work without having a higher rate of oxygen and heart beat. If you eat the above foods and nuts daily you would have enough of all minerals needed.

8.   Daily Consume Diets made up of 90% - 95% of Fruits and Vegetables

It is recommended by experts that your daily meal should be made up of about 90% to 95% of fruits and vegetables. Eat dark green vegetables daily.

Take oranges, apple, guava, paw-paw, pineapple, etc., daily.

9.   Avoid Harmful Habits Like Smoking, Caffeine, and Alcohol Intake.

 The entire habits above are harmful to your health. It is even stated clearly in cigarette packs, that tobacco smoking is dangerous and that smokers may die young. You must quit smoking to look 20 years younger.

Avoid caffeine and alcohol. As they contain harmful active components that are dangerous to health.

10.   Manage or Reduce Your Stress Level

Stress is sometimes brought about by fear, worry, anxiety, and anger. These things drain your energy, leaving you tired, haggard, and looking old. Learn to be quiet and relax well. Avoid tension or tense conditions.

11. Drink at least Eight to Ten Glasses of Water Daily

Drinking up to eight glasses of water daily would help keep you hydrated. Dehydration, will cause you to look old and worn out.

You can start with two glasses of water in the morning immediately you wake up from bed, and one glass before and after each three meals of a day.

If you do not eat three meals a day, you can still work it out. Water will also keep hunger pangs away from you.

12. Take Snacks Between Meals if Necessary

You can snack on some fruit when you feel like eating between meals, to help feel your stomach and reduce hunger pangs. Instead of snacking on biscuits, cakes, and other pastries, snack on fruits and little of yoghurt and nuts.

13. Do Medical Check-up

If you have anaemia or any body weakness, consult a doctor and make sure

that your blood is diagnosed to find out underlying causes of anaemia or any

other disease plaguing you, and to find cure or take all necessary

medication to rejuvenate your body. This will enable you to be healthy and

look younger.

2. Ways to Restore Your Skin to Perfect Beauty

The following information on ways to restore your skin to its perfect beauty can bring out best outlook and youthfulness, when undertaken appropriately.

In looking good through attaining and maintaining a beautiful skin, you need to put in effort to achieve this feat by following the under listed ways, to restore your skin to perfect beauty.

1.   Use Moisturising Soaks to Soothe Dryness

Get a winter sunflower bath by compounding ¼ cup shelled, unsalted sunflower seed; ½ teaspoon ground cinnamon; ¼ teaspoon ground nutmeg; and ½ teaspoon vitamin E oil.

Make a fine powder of sunflower seeds and oatmeal in a food processor, add the spices and oil. Add ¼ cup of mixture in your bath and soak for at least 20 minutes. This will help soothe, soften, and moisturise dry skin.

2.   Treat Your dry Skin with Honey

Honey can be used as a natural oil free moisturizer. It pulls and attaches water to the skin. In dry or combination complexions, mix two tablespoonfuls with two teaspoon of water, and massage into your face for three minutes, then rinse.

If you have oily skin, blend a tablespoon each of honey and lemon juice, leave on skin for three minutes and rinse. For a gentle facial scrub, mix equal parts of honey and cooked oatmeal.

3.   Avoid Picking at pimples if they Appear

You must avoid the temptation to pick or squeeze at your pimples if you have them. This action can cause the spread of bacteria and further infect the pore, leading to scarring.

4.   Avoid Using Hot Water on Your Face

Hot water affects the face negatively, by removing the natural oils that retain moisture and protect your skin. It also brings about conditions that require gentle care, such as inflamed capillaries and Rosales.

You can use facial cleansers with lukewarm water, two times a day. Avoid over washing your face to avoid skin sensitivity.

15

5.   Contact a Dermatologist for help

To avoid break outs that become much harder to cure, you need to see a dermatologist. You may be given oral prescription drugs and topical creams to control pimples and blackheads.

Seeing a dermatologist can also help you to know exactly what your condition is and avoid mistreatments that may worsen your skin condition.

Pamper your skin with a good lotion and the above ways to restore your skin to perfect beauty, and you shall look good.

How to Have a Smooth and Beautiful Skin

This information is designed to enable you know how to have a smooth skin, in such simple steps as never imagined, giving you that expected look of beauty and youthfulness..

Achieving a smooth skin involves carrying out daily routines that are geared towards building up your skin to the smoothness level you desire.

The following steps should be taken seriously on a daily basis, in order to give your skin that treatment required to enable your skin become smooth and good looking, to the admiration of all.

1. Drink 2 Glasses of Water First Thing in the Morning

Water is good for your body. You should train your body to be able to take in two glasses of water first thing in the morning. You may start with one glass first thing each morning and move to two glasses first thing each morning.

2. Drink 8 – 10 Glasses of Water Daily

Water is a major constituent of the human body. The human body is made up of 60 to 70% water. Water plays many import roles in the body, which include regulation of body temperature, transport of oxygen to various cells, expulsion of waste products, and protection of body organs, bones and joints.

Drinking eight to ten glasses of water daily will help flush your system of impurities and keep your body hydrated. We are made to understand that dehydration of the body is a major reason for various sicknesses that attack the body.

Never allow your body to become dehydrated. This is so, when you become thirsty and panting for water. This can injure your system.

In trying to achieve drinking 8 – to 10 glasses of water daily, drink one or two glasses first thing in the morning, one glass at 30 minutes or one hour after breakfast, one glass 30 minutes or one hour before lunch or 30 minutes/ 1hour after lunch.

You should also drink one glass 30 minutes or one hour before or after dinner. The remaining four to six glasses of water should be taken in between meals, before or after.

Your body cannot absorb large volumes of water at a moment, so drink little by little to attain the eight to ten glasses of water per day goal.

3.   Eat Diets of Mainly 90 Percent Fruits Daily

Learn to eat fruits daily, to treat your skin to that desired beauty and smoothness. Always eat fruits before meals on an empty stomach. Never eat fruit after meals, this will lead to bloating and bring about many health problems.

Note that whole fruit eating is better than drinking fruit juice. This is so, because whole fruits constitute fibre which is good for your body, as a cleanser and purifier of your body.

Your body will do better, look good, smooth, and beautiful when you take a fruit fast of one, three, or seven days.

4.   Engage in Physical Exercise Daily

Physical Exercise is needed by your body daily. Physical exercise will help keep your body fit and give your body the needed circulation required to nourish your body.

When you exercise, you lubricate your joints, clear your skin pores of blockages, keep you agile, strong, and healthy looking. Exercise will in turn cause your skin to flourish and look smooth.

Start engaging in brisk walking, jogging, swimming, running, stretching, and deep breathing, etc, to nourish your skin and look good.

5.   Sleep 8 Hours Daily

Sleep is good for your skin and general health. You would become restless and ill looking, if you deprive your self of needed sleep daily. Sleep will rejuvenate you body and help your skin look smooth and beautiful.

So, endeavour to sleep up to eight hours daily to better your health and skin.

6.   Use a Good Skin Moisturizer

Daily make use of a good moisturizing lotion to help condition your skin to perfect beauty and smoothness.

Daily application of the above how to tips will help your skin become smooth. Start taking small steps today towards your goal of having a smooth skin, and you would not be disappointed.

3.   Ways to Get Rid of Facial Pimples

This chapter provides information on facial spots and pimples, and also presents possible steps to enable you get rid of these conditions.

Pimples and facial spots are annoying inflammatory reactions due to the production of certain acids caused by abnormal response of some hormones circulating in the blood.

This leads to an increase production of sebum (an oily substance). Facial spots do not only affect youths, but can hang on to about 50 years of age.

To get rid of facial spots and pimples, the following steps or tips can help:

1. Drink More Water Daily

Water would help to free the hair roots of the clogging oil and thus reduce oil on the face or skin. So, drink a lot of water daily, up to about two litres. Do this and your face would clear within weeks.

2. Avoid a Stressful life

Stress causes over activity of the body chemicals or hormones, which result in facial pimples and spots.

3. Avoid Junk Foods

Avoid fried foods, cake, sweets, pastries, and too much chocolate, they cause pimples and facial spots to form and continue. Get a chocolate free diet.

4. Live in Ventilated Rooms with Fresh Air

Fresh air is good for your skin. Get fresh air indoors and outdoors.

5. Eat Balanced Diets

Eat meat, eggs, fish, cheese, milk, fruits and vegetables. They would keep your skin rejuvenated.

6. Put a Face Mask Weekly

Research the one that is best for you. For facial spots, apply lemon juice with cotton bud, to fight against bacteria.

7. Do Not Touch or Pick Your Spots and Pimples

Picking on spots and pimples, causes them to spread. So, do not squeeze the spots, do not cover with make-ups, and do not touch with your fingers

8. Avoid Worry and Anxiety

Worry aggravates the pimples and spots. Just concentrate on good things, and they shall surely clear away.

9. Get Plenty of Rest and Sleep

Sleep for eight hours daily, and give your body the needed rest.

10. Do Regular Face Washing

Wash your face with water and mild soap for about two to four times a day or every three hours. Do not use sponge.

Following the above cures brings relief and clears your face of the pimples and facial spots.

4. Beauty and Immunity Boosting Foods That Fight Ageing

Here is provided information about some beauty foods and immunity boosting foods that fight wrinkles, smoothens the skin, give healthy eyes, and drives cold and flu.

Eating special foods is a must for those who want to look younger and beautiful. When looking for such foods, beauty and immunity boosting foods should come readily in mind. The following beauty foods are also able to build up the muscles and burn of fats in the body:

1. Sweet potatoes - Smooths your skin

This vegetable is packed full with beauty boosting antioxidant, called beta carotene. When you consume sweet potatoes, your body works on the beta carotene and convert it to vitamin A, which then keeps your skin to be silky smooth.

A serving of sweet potatoes provides a double dose of vitamin A needs and has more than 10,000mg of beta carotene, which researchers say is linked to sun damage protection.

2. Blueberries - Fights wrinkles

The garnish, blueberries, in your morning oatmeal, can help to lower the signs of ageing, with high antioxidant content, vitamin C and E in particular, which strengthens collagen formation by reducing harmful free radical damage.

Report has it that researches at the United States Department of Agriculture (USDA) have found that a serving of blueberries gives the most antioxidants when compared to other fruits and vegetables.

It is recommended that you blend it and toss half a cup of blueberries into
your shakes.

3. Spinach - gives good eye health

It is reported that most people depended on spinach for muscle strength,
and that eating spinach is a major reason why many people do not need
eyeglasses.

Also, that according to USDA, one cup of cooked spinach gives the highest
amount of lutein and zeaxanthin, the antioxidants, most known for
preventing vision loss among vegetables.

Experts say that boosting your daily diet with a lutein-rich foods, such as
spinach, may help save your eyesight if you stay all day in front of your
computer.

28

It is recommended that you add olive oil, garlic, and lemon juice, and cook for two minutes.

4. Mushrooms

It is recommended that you toss in mushrooms. Mushrooms, according to research, are said to contain a type of sugar, with potent antiviral and antibacterial properties.

5. Salmon

It is reported that salmon contain lean protein that fights diseases, and also has good fats that help strengthen cell membranes, which help to speed up any healing time.

6. Pumpkin and other Leafy vegetables

These vegetables contain photochemical plant compounds that fight

disease-causing free radicals.

7. Garlic

Garlic is a natural germ fighter. It is made up of an antibacterial compound.

Research has it that this helps to stimulate white blood cells involved in

immunity work. It is recommended that you take two raw gloves of garlic

daily.

5. Ways to Flatten Your Tummy and Look Younger

Living a life with a bloated tummy portrays one as having no knowledge of what to do, in order to avoid, flatten, or control one's stomach. Though many things may result in a bloated tummy, there are simple ways in which one can use to flatten his or her stomach, in order to remain or look younger.

These simple ways are as follows:

1. Drink 8 – 10 Glasses of Water Daily.

Drinking lots of water daily would help to flush your system of clogs and impurities. So, drink lots of water daily, up to 8 – 10 glasses.

Drinking much water daily, would make you to eat less food. This is so because; the water would reduce hunger pangs, which would have caused you to eat much.

31

Much water helps in digestion, thereby removing the problem of a bloated tummy. Lots of water taken daily would help to flush any bloating your experience.

2. Avoid or Stop the intake of Alcohol.

Alcohol is dangerous to your health. Medical report say that alcohol causes bloating of tummy, due to its ability to cause the accumulation of fat in the stomach, by raising cortisol levels in the body.

Alcohol is also known to dehydrate the body, leaving patches of bloats in the tummy.

3. Consume More Fibre Daily.

Fibre in your diets would help prevent bloating due to constipation. Fibre diets also help to reduce your weight, including tummy weight gain. Cut down your intake of carbohydrates, such as white bread and white rice. To get fibre you need to take vegetables, fruits, brown, and whole wheat bread.

4. Eat Balanced and Small Portions of Food or Meals.

Eat small portions of food or meals throughout the day, than eating 2 - 3 big portions. Smaller portions eaten many times a day would help digestion to take place faster, to avoid giving your tummy a bloated look.

Eat healthy snacks like almonds every morning and night, which help in burning fat, and sometimes take desserts. All these will help to flatten your tummy.

Consume calcium diets or take it as a daily supplement of 1000mg to 1200mg. This would help keep your bones strong, and avoid fractured bones that cause slump looks. Avoid much intake of whole milk, it causes bloating of the tummy.

5. Engage in Daily Regular Exercise.

Exercise for 30 minutes to one hour indoors and 30 minutes to one hour outdoor daily or five times a week. Go jogging, swimming, brisk walking, and running. Do weight lifting, bench press to build your chest, and practice perfect posture exercises.

Also, always sit and stand straight. Never slump when sitting down. Be active daily. Exercise would help your system to be able to burn fat faster, thereby eliminating the problem of a bloated tummy.

6. Do Deep Breathing Daily.

Make sure that you do deep breathing for about 5 minutes daily. This should involve breathing from your abdomen, and not from your chest.

So, try to take the deep breath from your lower abdomen. This would help to pull your tummy back and help the burning of fat.

7. Avoid a stressful Life.

Medical report say that too much of stress results in increases in levels of a hormone, called cortisol levels, thus enabling fat to be sent to the stomach.

You must manage stress appropriately. Learn to rest well and eliminate stressful activities.

8. Quit or Stop Smoking.

As in stress, smoking is also reported to raise levels of cortisol. This causes smokers to have increases in abdominal fat, thus a bloated tummy.

As you seek to flatten your tummy, do not give up easily, just follow the above tips, and you shall get a flattened tummy that gives you fitness and a younger look you desire.

6. Get in Shape through Daily Exercise

This heading provides information on ways to get in shape through a regular program of daily exercise.

Daily exercise is necessary for you to be productive, lively, agile, and healthy. So, daily move your whole body for energy needed, by finding and abiding to certain exercises you cherish and enjoy. The following guides would do you good:

1. Select activities you enjoy partaking throughout the year.

Activities abound that can change your life. So, try and find activities that you can engage in throughout the year, like swimming and skiing in their proper season. Participate in activities that are enriching and live giving.

2.   Set Goals for Exercise

Set exercise goals for long term and short term. Your goal can be to engage in jogging every day and to walk briskly every day. Your reasons for exercising can also be stated to help you stay focused. With time your goal of getting in shape through exercise shall be attained.

3.   Let your muscles make your strong

You can exercise outdoors and indoors to keep fit and get in shape. But you can still do so indoors by using the sitting room or staircase to jog, jump, lift weights, stretching your body and run around, etc.

4.   Chose an appropriate time for your exercise

You can get in shape through exercise by keeping to the right time to exercise daily. Chose a time that you will be free from distraction from other activities that may try to rob you of your exercise. Once this is done, stick to it. It may be 7.00am or 6.00am or as desired.

5.   Join a fitness class to get monitored

A fitness class will help put you on a different footing altogether, where you get the best from trained personnel.

6.   Exercise with others

Exercising with others will help you learn from those who know more than you and also get the excitement of togetherness.

As you exercise on a daily basis and regularly, you will definitely get in

shape, and look healthy.

7. Say Bye to Grave Dangers of Smoking

Cigarette smokers may feel high and on top of the world, whenever they smoke, and thereby get grave dangers of smoking.

Tobacco is the most single avoidable health hazard today in the world. Statistics has it that tobacco is the cause of about 3000,000 deaths in America, on a yearly basis, mainly from cancer and heart diseases.

This is in addition to the halitosis, the stained fingers and teeth, the foul-smelling clothes, the smoker's cough, pains, and suffering.

Many health risk abound to smokers as compared to non-smokers. A smoker may say cigarette relaxes me in times of stress. Such must consider also the vulnerability of cancer of the bladder to which cigarette smoking brings.

How is it that cigarette smoking brings in such chronic sicknesses and even deaths. It happens that the respiratory tract of the lungs has lining of tiny hairs that help to flush out any mucus and foreign matter in the bronchi up to the throat, to be spit out through the mouth. Inhaling tobacco causes these little tiny hairs to become paralysed.

But while asleep and not smoking these cilia begin to recover, all through the night they stand up pushing upward, all the junk of tobacco. In the morning that is what you cough off with the familiar smokers cough.

After smoking for years, your powerful working cilia become totally destroyed, and never able to rise up again at night to try and perform their function of throwing or pushing up junk.

With this development, the mucus that have trapped pollutants, dust, tobacco junk, and foreign matter that you have inhaled, being accumulated, just deposits and remains there, instead of being pushed up and out.

These deposits become the breeding ground of bacteria and viruses, leading to colds, chronic bronchitis, respiratory infections, and other chronic diseases.

Smoking cigarette also brings about a disease in which the lung is less elastic, destroying the alveoli and air sacs that permit the exchange of oxygen for carbon dioxide. Then will lung cancer arise, in which statistics has it that eighty five percent of lung cancer cases are in men, and seventy five percent in women are connected to smoking cigarette. Cigarette smoking is a major cause of cancer death.

When a cigarette smoker inhales and drags the cigarette smoke into his or her lungs, poisonous gases and compounds, including cyanide, carbon monoxide, and volatile aromatic hydrocarbons.

The poisonous gases and compounds enter the bloodstream and go straight to the heart. Within seven seconds, the nicotine is pumped from the heart to brain, where it is absorbed.

Absorption of nicotine triggers the release of substances called, catecholamine, which produce adrenaline-like effect, increasing the heart rate and blood pressure. This makes smokers to feel high.

Smoking is an addiction that though difficult to quit, need be abandoned. This will save your life all the heartache, heart diseases, and many other troubles.

But you can quit if you are willing. For where there is a will to quit smoking, there is certainly going to be a way to quit smoking. Therefore stop buying and stop smoking today, and your health and youthfulness is guaranteed.

8. Daily Beauty Routines

Nature's beauty must be guarded seriously in order to enhance and maintain it. Beauty enhancers or daily beauty routines that will help you become more beautiful and good looking, must be visited on a daily basis. These daily beauty routines include:

a. Physical Activity or Exercise

Every morning when you wake up, after your devotion God, the next thing is to undertake or engage in physical activity or exercise. There are various exercise workouts that you can get adapted to, such as stretching, jogging, jumping, boxing the air, running, bending to touch the toes, deep breathing, and massaging the face and body, etc.

You may search and find professionals who offer exercise or physical activity services, to help you attain maximum benefits and results. You can buy some exercising equipment like exercise ball, jump rope, dumbbells, stationary bicycle, etc.

b. Brush Your Teeth and Mouth

Use a good toothpaste and toothpaste to freshen and whiten your teeth. To have a good appetite and fresh breath, you need to do this before drinking water or eating.

c. Drink Two Glasses of Water

Make sure that you drink about two glasses of water, first thing every morning. This will help prepare your body for the day and at the same time give you the needed freshness in all parts of the body. You can start with one glass or cup of water, and graduate to two glasses or cups each morning.

Your body requires freshness, and consuming clean water daily is very important. Water will enable your body to remain hydrated and youthful.

d. Shave and Shower

Keeping fresh and younger daily entails that you shave with a shaving cream and sharp razor or just a sharp razor would do. Then shower using shampoo and toilet soap with natural ingredients that are likely to protect than harm the skin.

e. Wipe Face and Body Using a Clean Towel

Use a clean towel to wipe your body after showering, to avoid adding dirts to the already washed skin. Remove excess moisture in the hair using the towel.

46

f. Moisturize Your Skin Perfectly

To obtain best results, you must moisturize your face and body with immediately after showering or bath. Make use of moisturizer that would help glow your skin.

Get a tinted moisturizer to help glow your skin and make you look younger and beautiful.

g. Brush, Comb or Style Your Hair

Use a good and sizeable brush or comb to set your hair to make you look good, and younger.

h. Wash Hands throughout the Day

Hand washing and use of hand sanitizers should be undertaken throughout the day, to ensure cleanliness and freedom from disease-causing agents.

i. Before Going to Bed at Night

You need to brush your teeth again / whitening application and shower at night . If you wish you could just wash your face with toilet soap or an oil-free wash, to refresh.

After showering or washing face, wipe face and body with a clean towel, before using moisturizing lotion on the skin and face.

j. Brush Your Nails to keep Them Neat

Wash and brush your toes and finger nails daily to keep them neat and

youthful. If need be cut them to keep them free from harbouring germ

underneath.

9. Ways to Minimize Your stress Level

Stress management begins with knowing the causes of stress in your life. Is it constant worry about work deadlines, procrastination, actual job demands, family demands, etc.

The following ways can help you to minimize your stress level:

a. Avoid smoking, alcohol drinking, overeating, under-eating, over sleeping, procrastination, and endless hours before your home screens like television.

b. Avoid Unnecessary Stress

Avoid engaging in stressful jobs for too long, and people who causes stress. You need reduce your stay before your television or computer that causes you stress.

c. Good Management of Time

Bad management of your time can cause stress.

d. Division of labour

Make sure that you do not do everything alone. You will be stressed, if you do so. Give or pay people to handle or do some jobs to avoid stress.

e. Change Your Attitudes and Some Things

Try and control what you can control and change some attitudes responsible for stress.

f. Learn to Forgive Others

Forgivenesses will help you keep away stress out of your life. Whatever wrong any might have done to you, forgivenesses is very important to stay free from being stress.

g. Spend Some Time Relaxing

Go for a walk, drink a cup of tea, snack on a fruit, listen to music, and go to the garden. Set aside time for relaxation in your life.

Do something you enjoy like playing piano, singing, and workout.

h. Laugh Often to Keep Fresh

i. Eat Balanced Diets

Nourish your body well. Start your day with breakfast, and keep your body youthful with balanced, nutritious and delicious meals throughout the day.

Avoid sugar and caffeine. They are harmful to your body functioning and youthfulness

j. Sleep well

You must learn to sleep well daily.

10. Proper Eating or Nutrition and Best Foods for Energy

Proper eating or nutrition and best foods for energy can help boost your youthfulness on a daily basis.

Food is the fuel of our body craves and eating the right type of food is very important, in order that we may keep our body strong and full of energy. If you desire to loss weight, eating small amount of food, and exercising regularly, can be help you to achieve the goal, in addition to other things.

The following guide will help you get the best out of proper eating and best energy foods, to enable you become younger than your age:

a. Consume the Right Type of Food

Consume grains, fruits, and vegetables regularly. Also, make sure that you stay away from fried foods or fatty foods. Consume up to four or five small meals, rather than one or two large bowls. Try not to miss or skip breakfast or other meals, so that your body system will function normally. Avoid junk foods, like cakes, sweets, and fast foods.

b. Eat high energy foods daily to keep you on the go.

Your stress level can be managed or reduced with regular and daily consumption of high energy foods. The following are best high energy foods.

i. Oatmeal

Oatmeal is a source of fibre. Fibre has the ability to help your digestion, so that you body can have a steady flow of energy as carbohydrate enters into your blood system. Eating fibre means eating the right type of food.

ii. Beans

Beans aid the problem of low iron deficiency which brings the problem of sluggishness. Best is best eaten when prepared as soup.

iii. Snack Banana

Bananas contain potassium, a mineral element that help in nerves and muscles normal functioning.

iv. Green Spinach

Green spinach contains the magnesium mineral. Consuming spinach ensures that you are taking in adequate levels of the mineral.

v. Strawberries

Strawberries can aid your body to absorb iron, because it contains vitamin C.

vi. Soy bean Products

Soy beans have many health benefits and contain calcium. It can be consume as soy milk, and other products.

vii. Other high energy foods include tuna, whole grain bagels, and low-fat yoghurt.

Going raw is preferred to cooked food, because what your body need is often destroyed through cooking. It is best to go 100% natural with no supplements, to help make you younger looking and with a beautiful skin.

c. Drink Water Daily and Regularly

Water is very important for our body's well-being. Water helps in digestion of food in the body, and keeps the body and skin in optimal conditions. It is recommended that you take eight to ten glasses of water daily. You can start with 2 glasses of water, first thing in the morning.

Work out your proper eating and use of best foods for energy, for good health and a better skin.

11. Protect Your Skin From Exposure to Sun

The sun can cause damage to your skin thereby causing you sun burn, dryness, or other exposure effects.

You can help avoid skin cancer and wrinkles as you give attention to protecting your skin from sun rays exposure.

The following ways would help you get protection from sun rays:

a. Wear Sunshade Caps and Glasses

Ultraviolet rays can damage your skin fast, therefore protect yourself through the use of face cap and sunshade glasses. Wear sunglasses that protect sides of your eyes.

b. Avoid Sun Bathing

Sun bathing can cause damage to your skin. Stay away from sun tanning activities.

c. Avoid Total Exposure to Sunlight

When sunlight is most intense, you need to avoid total exposure from 10 am. to 4 pm. During intense sunlight period, dwell in shade places.

d . Wear Protective Clothing

Wear clothes that cover your skin, including legs and hands. With these protective clothing, you can still expose yourself to sunlight but with reduced exposure.

If you can start today to observe and do the above, you would be happy, as you start seeing yourself looking 20 years younger than your age.

To your younger looking success.

I